All About Menopause

Dr. Sheila Harrison

Disclaimer

This content serves to provide general information about the disease and aims to empower you to seek prompt medical assistance if necessary to prevent complications. It's essential to stress that this information is not a substitute for consulting a qualified physician. The field of medical science is continually evolving, and due to the dynamic nature of medical knowledge, we recommend seeking expert advice if you encounter any inconsistencies or intend to take action based on the information in this content. Never disregard professional medical guidance or delay treatment based on something you've read online, including this material, or from any other online source. Always remember that the internet cannot cure you; rather, healing comes through the guidance of medical professionals and the providence of God.

Table of Contents

Overview

Menopause is the end of the menstrual cycle. It affects a woman's reproductive system and is a universal and permanent aspect of aging generally. After 12 months of amenorrhea, menopause is identified. Menopause is characterized by a wide range of symptoms, such as irregular or unpredictable menses; vasomotor and urogenital symptoms like dyspareunia and vaginal dryness; and problems with mood and sleep.

Before and right after menopause, there are hormonal shifts and accompanying clinical symptoms. Although the menopausal transition (MT), a more modern term, is increasingly being used to refer to this era, it is still often known as the climacteric or perimenopause. Typically, the MT starts years before menopause.

There is a simultaneous and ongoing growth in the proportion of middle-aged and older people as well as women who spend the majority of their life in a hypoestrogenic state (Hypoestrogenism, or estrogen deficiency, refers to a lower than normal level of estrogen. It is an umbrella term used to describe estrogen deficiency in various conditions). An increasing number of women will face the effects of gonadal steroid hormone depletion and live to be around 79 years of age.

While the duration of menopause has extended to up to one-third of the life cycle, the average age at which menopause occurs has remained constant throughout antiquity, at roughly 50–51 years. Menopause struck women in ancient Greece at the same age as it does today, with the onset of symptoms typically occurring between 45.5 and 47.5 years of age.

Section 1

What is Menopause?

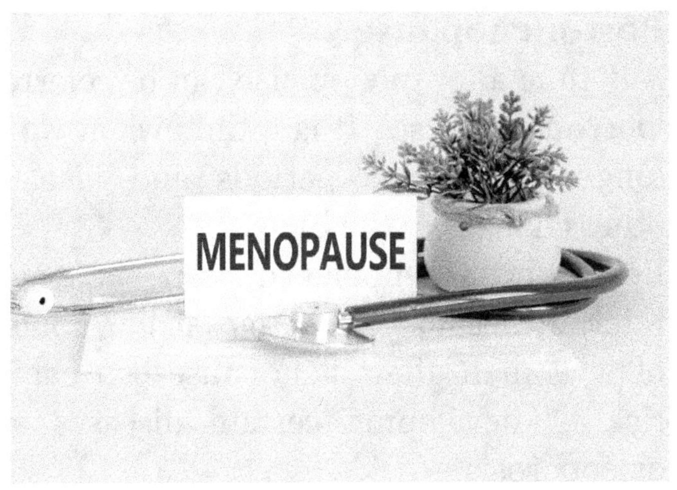

Menopause is a time of natural female hormonal changes, most notably, the end of menstruation. It happens gradually over a period of months or years, starting with irregular periods and often accompanied by other symptoms like hot flushes and sleeplessness.

Perimenopause

Peri- means 'around', and so 'perimenopause' refers to the time period around menopause. It can be used to describe the time from the first suspected symptoms (or erratic periods) up until the end of menopause (i.e. 12 months after the final period).

Post-menopause

Any time after menopause can be referred to as 'post-menopause'. It is a time when women no longer experience periods and also heralds other changes in the body.

Being post-menopausal can be medically relevant because the different hormone profile of a woman after menopause can change her risk of developing certain diseases such as osteoporosis.

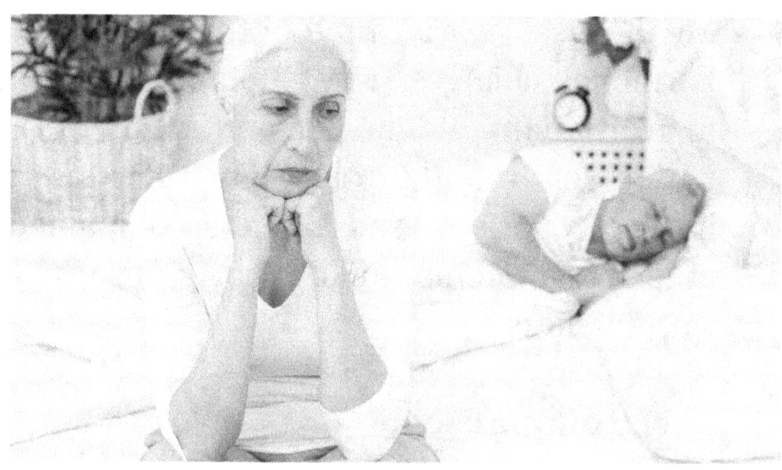

Section 2

At What Age Does Menopause Start?

Menopause usually occurs in the late forties or early fifties. If menopause begins before the age of 40, it is referred to as **'Early Menopause'** or **'Premature Menopause'**. There is a range of genetic and environmental factors which also seem to influence the age at which women usually experience menopause, and lots of women begin menopause at around the same age their own mothers did.

Early Menopause / Premature Menopause

With the changing lifestyle, the incidence of early menopause may have seen an increase in numbers. Since menopause is a very important part of women's health, early menopause can have serious impacts.

What is early menopause?

In menopause, a woman's ovaries stop functioning and producing hormones and eggs. Gradually, periods also stop. The average age for normal menopause is 51 years. We call it early menopause when someone has it before the age of 45 years. We have another category called premature menopause. In this, a woman gets menopause before the age of 40. It is not uncommon but we do see patients with either premature or early menopause.

What are the potential causes of early menopause?

The age of 51 is now considered normal for menopause. A few years back, 45 years was thought to be the normal age for menopause. But with drastic changes in lifestyle, the age is changing.

However, apart from lifestyle, few other factors like:

- Diet
- **Smoking:** Smoking can be the reason behind the increase in the cases of early menopause too. Smoking is a big risk factor,

but lifestyle in my opinion doesn't affect it so much.

- **Genetic predisposition:** A genetic predisposition means that there is an increased chance that a person will develop a disease based on their genetic makeup.,

- **Endocrinological Disorder:** An endocrine disorder results from the improper function of the endocrine system, which includes the glands that secrete hormones, the receptors that respond to hormones and the organs that are directly impacted by hormones. At any one of these points, dysfunction can occur and cause wide-ranging effects on the body..

- **Oophorectomy**: Surgery to remove ovaries or Treatment for cancer in the pelvic area can cause early menopause.

- **Hysterectomy:** a surgical operation to remove all or part of the uterus.

- **Fragile X carrier:** A fragile X carrier is someone who has an altered FMR1 gene(The *FMR1* gene provides instructions for making a protein called FMRP. This protein is present in many tissues, including the brain, testes, and ovaries), but does not show any obvious signs or symptoms of fragile X

syndrome. Women who are fragile X carriers have up to a 50 percent chance of having a child with fragile X syndrome.
- **Autoimmune disorders:** An autoimmune disorder occurs when the body's immune system attacks and destroys healthy body tissue by mistake
- **Living at high altitude**
- History of receiving certain chemotherapy medications or undergoing radiotherapy

Are there any long-term health risks associated with early menopause?

Females have a hormone called estrogen which is normally produced by the ovaries and is a very important hormone for a female body. Once a person reaches menopause, estrogen production reduces. As a result of this, they can get osteoporosis, heart disease, skin problems, hair problems, etc.

If you get your menopause at the right age, your body gradually gets to the menopausal phase, and still, you may get these issues sometimes. However, if you have early menopause, you have a higher chance of getting these problems in the future.

What are the signs and symptoms of early menopause and how do we diagnose it?

Firstly, females will start experiencing menstrual irregularities. They may have only spotting during the menses. This is the first sign of menopause. So, when a patient goes for a check-up or an ultrasound by which doctors can detect that the ovaries are smaller than what they are expected to be. Then they may do other hormonal tests for the hormones called FSH and LH to confirm this. If their findings confirm their suspicion of menopause, they may repeat the tests after a month and finalize confirmation of the diagnosis. Apart from this, a female may experience hot flashes, night sweats, etc., which is not normal for a younger female. Therefore, if these symptoms are there along with irregular periods, it may be early menopause.

What is the treatment process for early menopause?

In most of the patients with early or premature menopause, we probably have to give hormone replacement therapy (HRT). Although it is very safe these days as we have low-dose hormones, I don't immediately jump to HRT as a treatment. I ask them to follow a healthier lifestyle with a healthy diet increasing the consumption of soya products and milk products, exercise, etc. If the symptoms continue, then we have to put them on HRT.

Are there any preventive measures to reduce the risk of early menopause? As I already mentioned, smoking is a huge risk factor. So, people can avoid it as a preventive measure against early menopause. If someone has a family history of menopause, we cannot prevent it but we can be aware of it. The moment you feel that you may be having menopausal symptoms, you can go to a gynecologist so that a treatment like HRT can be started well in time. Nobody can prevent menopause. We can only treat the symptoms and other problems that are associated with menopause.

Section 3

Why does Menopause Happen?

As we get older, our reproductive cycle slows down. Ovaries start to produce less oestrogen, which affects the menstrual cycle. This explains why the menstrual cycle starts to become irregular. Menopause then marks the time when women are no longer able to bear children naturally.

Interestingly, post-menopausal women with healthy uteruses (wombs) can still become pregnant through in vitro fertilization. There are numerous examples of women acting as surrogates.

Sometimes, menopause may happen earlier due to an operation to remove the ovaries (oophorectomy), a medical condition, chemotherapy, or radiotherapy which affects the ovaries' oestrogen production.

A hysterectomy (removal of the womb) for a condition like uterine or cervical cancer may or may not also involve the removal of ovaries. If the ovaries are removed, menopause begins immediately. If the ovaries are left intact and in situ, they continue to produce oestrogen and so menopause does not begin. On average, however, women who have had a hysterectomy without oophorectomy still tend to begin menopause slightly earlier than women who have not had a hysterectomy.

Section 4

Signs & Symptoms of Menopause

The experiences of menopause can vary widely from one person to the next, but there are some symptoms that are common throughout menopause.

Physical Signs/Effects

- **Hot Flushes or Hot Flashes:**One of the most common symptoms of menopause is 'hot flush' or 'hot flash'. This refers to a sudden feeling of warmth or extreme heat, sometimes with sweating and skin flushing. This feeling can last for several minutes or even up to an hour. The frequency and intensity of hot flushes vary depending on the individual. Some people may experience hot flushes several times a day while for others, hot flushes are only occasional. They can be relatively mild or very uncomfortable.

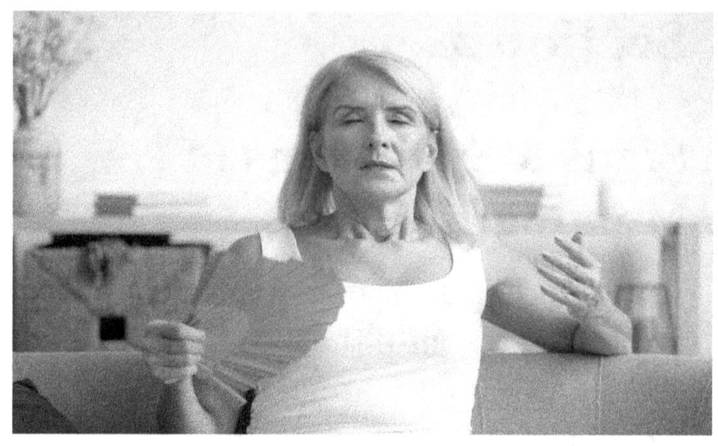

- **Sleep Disturbance:** A combination of hormonal changes, hot flushes and other symptoms of menopause can result in sleep problems. Depending on the individual and the underlying cause of insomnia, different people may have different ways to manage it. However, it is important to find a way to get quality sleep as sleeplessness can have a serious impact on other areas of life. If you are experiencing severe insomnia, it would be best to consult a doctor and work out a solution together.

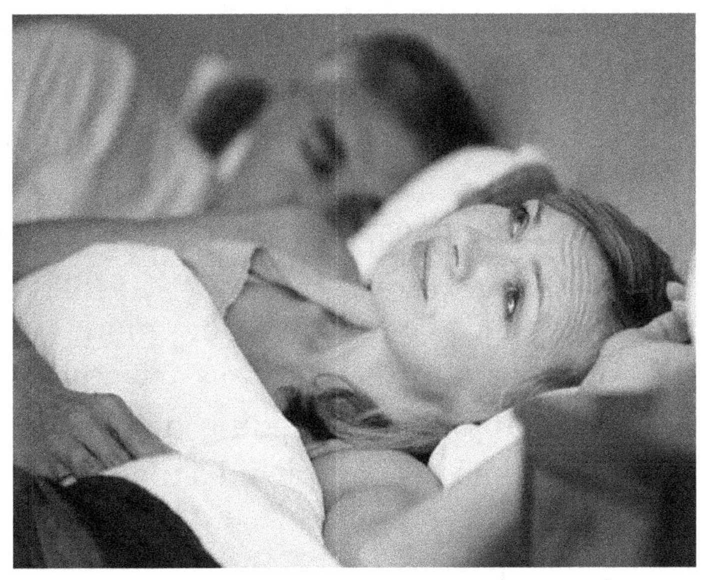

- **Mood Changes:** Besides hormonal changes, there are many other aspects of menopause that can affect mood too. Menopause often coincides with a time of change in family circumstances and position; children growing up and leaving home, perhaps having children of their own. During this time of physical and emotional changes, it's normal to have mixed feelings. This can affect mood and emotional resilience, and – although it's normal – it is okay to need support through this time.

- **Irregular Periods or Spotting:** Menopause is not over until 12 months after the last episode of bleeding, and menstrual bleeding can be very erratic peri-menopause. Some people go months between periods, while others may experience occasional or more frequent spotting. Any worrying symptoms like unusually heavy bleeding or bleeding after menopause is completed should be checked out by a GP as it could indicate other problems.

- **Problems with Sex:** Intercourse can be trickier after menopause as vaginal dryness often becomes an issue. Mood swings, tiredness, and hormonal changes can also affect libido. However, many women do still have a happy and active sex life after menopause with the help of products such as simple lubricants or medicated preparations containing estrogen.

- **Changes in Appearance of the Skin:** The appearance of the skin changes during menopause due to a reduced amount of collagen in the skin. Collagen is the substance that keeps our skin taut and springy. With less collagen, we develop more visible wrinkles and parts of our body begin to sag.

- **Changes to the Hair:** The way hair is distributed across our body is largely controlled by hormones, and so the hair on the head often starts to thin as hormone levels change through and after menopause. Some women also develop hair where they didn't have any before – often on the chin and around the mouth.

Clinical Signs/effects

During the menopausal transition, physiologic changes in responsiveness to gonadotropins and their secretions occur, with wide variations in hormone levels. Women often experience a range of symptoms clinically, including the following:
- Insomnia
- Weight gain and bloating
- Mastodynia
- Depression
- Headache

Section 5

Poor Sleep: The Lesser-Known Symptom of Menopause and Perimenopause

Sleep problems are a lesser-known symptom of menopause, compared to hot flushes and joint pain. Yet, it affects 35% to 60% of post-menopausal women and 39% to 47% of perimenopausal women. Could menopause be the cause of your poor sleep?

For women who have menopause and perimenopause, sleep problems are often an overlooked symptom. While sleeping issues are common during menopause, they can start in perimenopause. You may notice these symptoms:

- Hot flushes
- Mood swings
- Difficulty having intercourse due to vaginal dryness

- Sleep disorders, including insomnia, sleep-disturbed breathing, and restless leg syndrome
- Joint pain
- Fatigue
- Dry, itchy skin
- Hair loss
- Weight gain

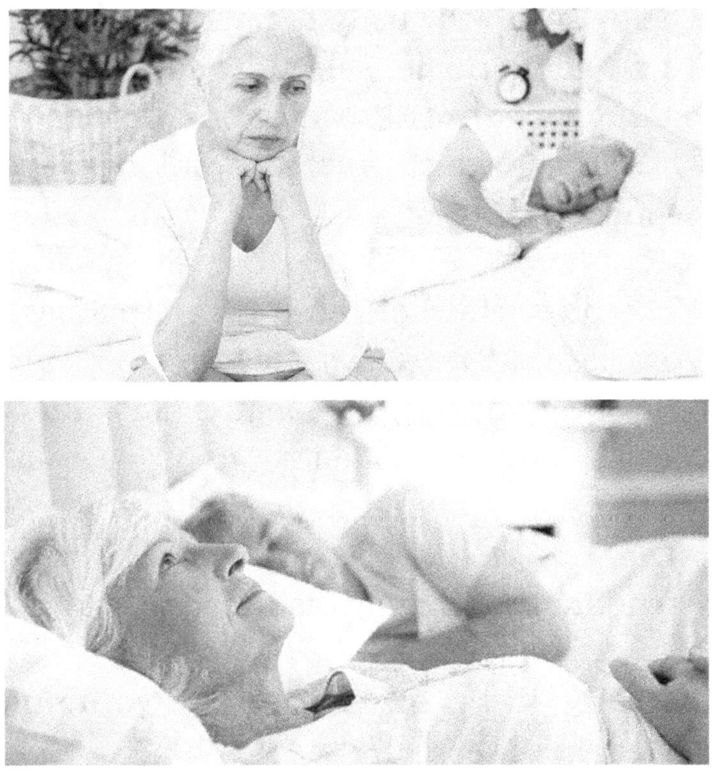

Sleep Disorders

Why Do Menopause Causes Sleep Problems

Fluctuating and decreasing estrogen and progesterone levels as a woman approaches menopause can cause sleep problems.

The two key female reproductive hormones, estrogen and progesterone, affect sleep quality. Estrogen influences your sleep-wake cycle, helps keep your body temperature low at night for comfortable sleep and is naturally anti-depressive. Progesterone affects proper breathing, which enables you to sleep more soundly.

The production of these two hormones in the ovaries fluctuates in the lead-up to menopause. However, during menopause and after, their levels are permanently lower because the ovaries stop producing them altogether.
The two stages of menopause share similar symptoms, including disturbed sleep.

TCM's View on Sleeping Problems and Menopause

In Traditional Chinese Medicine (TCM), women experience a depletion of Kidney *jing* (essence) and reproductive essence around the age of 49. This is when they're nearing menopause.

This depletion in Kidney *jing* leads to sleeping problems due to:

- A disruption in the balance between *yin* (cool, passive energy) and *yang* (warm, active energy) caused by Liver and Kidney *Yin* Deficiency. *Yang* energy remains high at night, causing insomnia.
- Disharmony of the Heart and Kidneys leads to Heart Fire and Kidney *Yin* Deficiency. This causes a "monkey mind" and a racing Heart, leading to dream-disturbed sleep.
- Liver *Qi* (vital life force) Stagnation leads to emotional disturbance as the Liver governs your emotions. This contributes to poor sleep quality. Women who experience this complain of anxiety that robs them of rest.

Western and TCM Treatment for Menopause and Sleep Problems

Doctors would usually recommend hormone replacement therapy (HRT) to replenish a decline in oestrogen levels. It can help relieve symptoms caused by the drop.

Meanwhile in TCM, treatments to ease symptoms of menopause and perimenopause involve herbal remedies and acupuncture.

Suriya recalls trying different ways to improve her sleep before turning to TCM. "I tried a lot of things. I ate healthily, exercised regularly, and did breathing exercises before bed."

"I lived in a city with a large population of people of East Asian ancestry, and I learned about TCM from one of my friends. I read up on the research and decided to try it too," she shares. Her TCM physician put her on a combination of herbal therapy, moxibustion, and acupuncture. After a few months, she noticed improved sleep and overall health. This gradual positive change has remained.

Section 6

How Is Menopause Diagnosed?

Menopause is diagnosed after 12 months of amenorrhea (An abnormal absence of menstruation).

Hormonal changes and clinical symptoms occur over a period leading up to and immediately following menopause; this period is frequently termed the climacteric or perimenopause but is increasingly referred to as the menopausal transition.

Usually, the symptoms alone are enough to make a diagnosis of menopause.

To confirm the diagnosis, blood or urine tests may be completed to show the fluctuating levels of hormones that happen around the time of menopause.

Menopause is only considered completed 12 months after the last menstrual period, so the end of menopause is only diagnosed retrospectively.

Although we talk about *'diagnosis'* and *'symptoms'* in medical terms, menopause is a natural and normal occurrence, rather than a medical condition. Many women do not have any trouble at all. On the other hand, some people experience severe symptoms which can affect their everyday life. Remember that everyone's experience is different and it is okay to seek professional advice and treatment for troublesome symptoms.

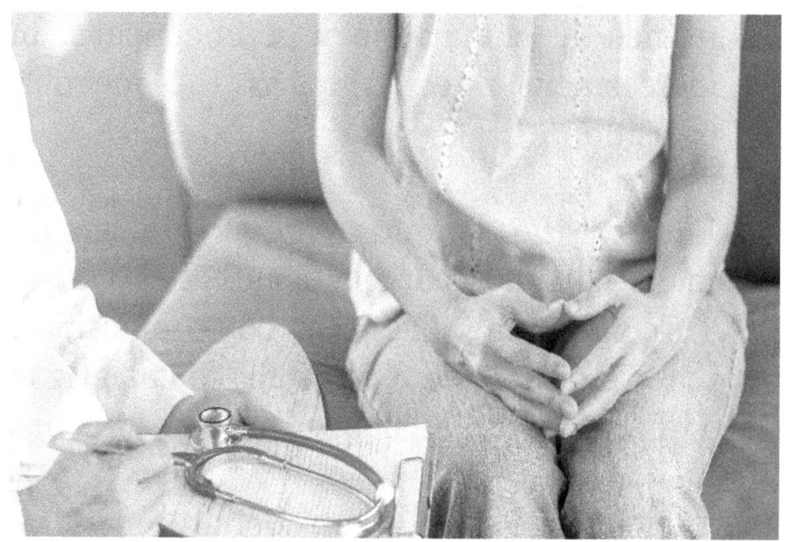

Section 7

How Long Do Menopause Symptoms Last?

Menopause lasts from the time the first symptoms begin – this may be when periods become erratic, or classic symptoms like hot flushes start to happen – to the date 12 months after the last period od a woman's life time. The average total length of menopause symptoms is more than seven years, and symptoms are reported to continue after the final menstrual period for around four and a half years.

However, it is important to note that everyone's experience is not the same, and may also be affected by treatment and management.

The temporal pattern of symptoms is as follows:
- Symptoms may begin up to 6 years before the final menstrual period and continue for a variable number of years after the final menstrual period.
- As the postmenopause years progress, with an accompanying loss of ovarian response

to gonadotropins, associated affective symptoms of menopause also decline
- On pelvic examination, the effects of gonadal hormone depletion (which may be noted before menopause in some women) are as follows:
- With loss of estrogen, the vaginal epithelium becomes redder as the epithelial layer thins and the small capillaries below the surface become more visible
- Later, as the vaginal epithelium further atrophies, the surface becomes pale because of a reduced number of capillaries
- Rugation diminishes, and the vaginal wall becomes smooth
- The menopausal ovary diminishes in size and . is no longer palpable during gynecologic examination
- The uterus becomes smaller
- Fibroids, if present, become less symptomatic, sometimes shrinking to the point where they can no longer be palpated on manual pelvic examination
- In older women, a general loss of pelvic muscle tone occurs, sometimes manifested as prolapse of reproductive or urinary tract organs

Urogenital effects of diminished hormone levels are as follows:
- A decrease in urine pH leading to a change in bacterial flora may result in pruritus and a malodorous discharge
- Vaginal changes often result in insertional dyspareunia
- Endometriosis and adenomyosis are alleviated
- Atrophic cystitis, when present, can mimic a urinary tract infection

Section 8

Clinical markers/Signature   Menopause

Laboratory markers

Laboratory markers of menopause include the following:

- An increase in serum follicle-stimulating hormone (FSH) and decreases in estradiol and inhibin are the major endocrine changes that occur during the transition to menopause

- FSH levels are higher than luteinizing hormone (LH) levels, and both rise to even higher values than those seen in the surge during the menstrual cycle

- The FSH rise precedes the LH rise; FSH is the diagnostic marker for ovarian failure, while LH is not necessary to make the diagnosis

- The large cyclical variation of estradiol and estrone observed during the menstrual years ceases, and fluctuation in levels is small and inconsequential, with the mean value being considerably lower

- No specific changes in thyroid function related to menopause have been found

Endometrial changes

- Endometrial biopsy can show a range of endometrial appearances, from mildly proliferate to atrophic

- No secretory changes are observed after menopause, because no ovulation occurs and therefore no corpus luteum forms to produce progesterone

Endometrial hyperplasia is a sign of hyperstimulation by estrogen from either endogenous sources or replacement therapy and may be a precursor of endometrial cancer. Endometrial hyperplasia can also be suggested by ultrasonographic findings (ie, endometrial thickness >5 mm), which are useful for excluding hyperplasia and cancer of the endometrium in postmenopausal women

Osteoporosis

Bone loss accelerates in the late menopausal transition and continues for the first few years after menopause. Postmenopausal women and elderly women should be treated early and on a long-term basis unless a contraindication to such treatment exists.

Current treatment options for preventing fractures among postmenopausal women with osteoporosis include the following:

- Bisphosphonates (alendronate, etidronate, ibandronate, risedronate, zoledronic acid)
- Selective estrogen receptor modulators (SERMs; eg, raloxifene)
- Calcium
- Vitamin D
- Calcitonin
- Monoclonal antibodies

Section 9

Menopause Treatment

The main reasons for treating symptoms of the menopausal transition and actual menopause are as follows:
- To provide relief of vasomotor symptoms
- To reduce the risk of unwanted pregnancy
- To avoid the irregularity of menstrual cycles
- To preserve bone
- To lower the risk of disease
- improve quality of life

If the symptoms of menopause are affecting your quality of life, there are several medical treatments that can be prescribed by a GP, as well as a range of alternative therapies and naturopathic remedies that may help.

Hormone Replacement Therapy (HRT): HRT replaces either oestrogen alone or estrogen and progesterone together. HRT can ease the symptoms of menopause. Some people find this treatment essential to get them through periods of severe symptoms. HRT is available in many forms, including tablets, patches that stick on the skin, and vaginal creams and pessaries. However, there are risks associated with some forms of HRT and it may not be recommended for those with a history of breast cancer.The treatment is associated with health risks such as blood clots, stroke, and dementia, among other issues. If you choose this route, your doctor will likely recommend the lowest possible dose.

Administration routes for hormone therapy are as follows:
- Oral
- Transdermal
- Topical
- Vaginal route cream, ring, or tablet for vaginal symptoms

Non Hormonal therapy: In June 2013, the FDA approved paroxetine mesylate (Brisdelle) as the first nonhormonal therapy for vasomotor symptoms (VMS) (hot flashes) associated with menopause.

Antidepressants: Antidepressants are often used to reduce the effect of mood changes and sleeplessness during menopause. Some antidepressants also have a beneficial effect on other menopause symptoms, including hot flushes. Besides managing the symptoms of menopause, women should also take note of the increased risks of certain conditions post-menopause. For example, reduced oestrogen production increases the risk of osteoporosis, and so it is important to take the necessary steps to manage this risk, such as using medication or supplements.

Menopause Supplements: There are lots of different supplements for menopausal and post-menopausal women. These range from herbal or homeopathic remedies to specially blended multivitamins. The evidence behind the supplements available is variable, so it is important to do some research before taking supplements. If in doubt, always turn to a medical professional for advice. Some of the most common herbal and alternative medicines marketed for managing menopause include:

- **Red Clover:** One of the most common herbal remedies used in menopause, red clover has been the subject of several studies to determine its effectiveness in reducing menopausal symptoms. The results have been variable, but show some promise.

- **Ginseng:** Research into ginseng in menopause has found that, while it does not seem to have a significant impact on troublesome hot flushes, it can help with depression and mood changes.
- **Evening Primrose Oil:** Evening primrose oil has been used for many years to reduce the intensity of hot flushes in menopause.
- **Black Cohosh:** Like evening primrose oil, black cohosh is used to reduce the intensity of hot flushes, and also seems to reduce its frequency as well.
- **Soy:** The phytoestrogens in some plants are thought to reduce the effects of fluctuating oestrogen in women's bodies during menopause. Soy can be incorporated into the diet in the form of soy milk, edamame beans, tofu, various meat or dairy alternatives, or concentrated supplements.

Taking a multivitamin designed for menopause is often recommended by healthcare professionals. While a healthy diet alone can provide a person with all the vitamins and minerals they need for good health, there may be some specific requirements during and after menopause.

Bone density decreases markedly after menopause so Calcium and vitamin D supplements are commonly recommended – alongside a good diet and exercise – to help prevent osteoporosis. The B vitamins, along with vitamins C and D are also particularly essential for menopause.

Acupuncture: Acupuncture, including auricular therapy (ear acupuncture), is another proven treatment for menopause-related sleep disturbances. "The emphasis is to nourish *yin* and suppress hyperactive *yang*, nourish the Heart and calm the spirit," Physician Lim explains.

Acupuncture requires sessions with a professionally trained and licensed acupuncturist. In the meantime, you can improve sleep by performing acupressure on yourself.

Section 10

Menopause Risk Factors

Disease risk

In the Women's Health Initiative (WHI), greater safety and possible benefit from hormone or estrogen therapy for women in their 50s, with potential harm for older women, were observed with respect to the following :
- Coronary artery disease (CAD)
- Total myocardial infarction
- Colorectal cancer
- Total mortality

Treatment/Medication Risk

Although immediate use of hormone or estrogen therapy in the early postmenopausal time may reduce the risk of CAD, the WHI clearly showed that women more than 9 years post menopause should not be started on hormone therapy or estrogen therapy for CAD prevention.

Contraindications for estrogen therapy include the following:
- Undiagnosed vaginal bleeding
- Severe liver disease
- Pregnancy
- Venous thrombosis
- Personal history of breast cancer

Well-differentiated and early endometrial cancer, once treatment for the malignancy is complete, is no longer an absolute contraindication. Progestins alone may relieve symptoms if the patient is unable to tolerate estrogens.

Section 11

Lifestyle Tips for Menopause Management

Many of the symptoms of menopause can be well managed using simple measures. For example, wearing cool clothing, having cold drinks on hand, and using fans or other cooling measures can help with hot flashes.

Post-menopause, being aware of the altered profile of disease risk is important. Staying active and following a healthy diet helps reduce the risk of cardiovascular disease, weight gain, and the conditions associated with a high body mass index (BMI) like type 2 diabetes and high blood pressure. A diet high in calcium and vitamin D can help maintain healthy bones into later life.

Continuing to attend regular health check-ups, breast screening, and taking prescribed medication as directed are all essential for staying healthy after menopause.

As we get older and face a higher risk of conditions associated with ageing, it is essential to maintain a healthy lifestyle to mitigate that risk. A healthy diet, regular exercise, and cutting back on caffeine and alcohol are a good start. If you smoke, quitting is also one of the most important things you can do to keep diseases at bay and ensure a healthy life.

* 9 7 9 8 8 6 7 5 7 5 8 0 9 *